The Definitive Guide of Intermittent Fasting

How to Benefit from Fasting and is it for Everyone

TABLE OF CONTENTS

CHAPTER ONE: What is Intermittent Fasting (IF)?

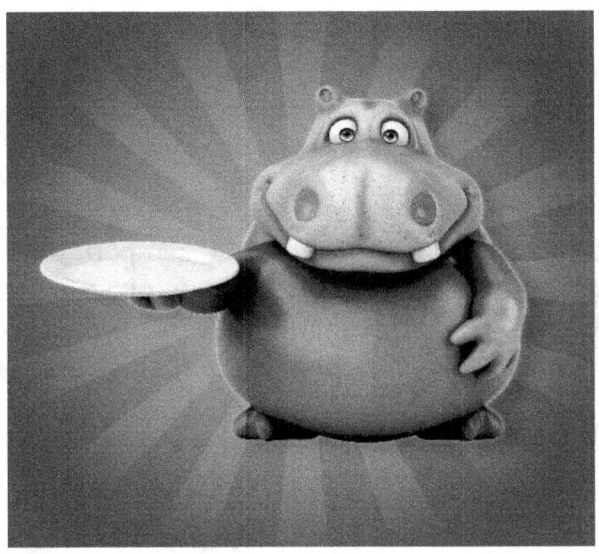

Excess foods are stored within the body either as glycogen or as fat for future use. The body requires time, therefore, to utilize them. For example, during the night when you sleep, you are in a state where your body utilizes the stored nutrients during the fasting period to maintain the normal body functioning.

This is the fasting period. The first meal we take when we wake tends to break your fast and hence the name breakfast. In addition to this, our bodies undergo states of fasting where they break down the foods to produce the necessary energy every time we are not eating. Because of this, it is now important to note that fasting is part of our daily life.

Unlike starvation, which involves the involuntary absence of food, fasting is the intentional withholding of foods for either health or spiritual among others reasons best known to the practitioners. This, therefore, means that one can decide when to start a fast as well as stopping it. The eating pattern that recycles between the fasting and feasting is what is now known as intermittent fasting. It focuses on when to eat rather than what to eat.

The main aim of fasting is to allow the body use the stored energy. With this in mind, it is important to avoid foods rich in calories. However, taking coffee, tea, and water among other non-caloric beverages is advisable when you are in the starvation mode. Due to the many forms of fasting, some types allow the intake of low-calorie foods. The different forms are explained in detail later in the book. During this hunger period, supplements are important provided there are no calories in them. This reenergizes the body. The water prevents the body against dehydration. Lack of enough nutrients in our diet would call for the substitution.

How intermittent fasting operates

It is important first to note that life is all about the balance. For example, a balance between the yin and the yang as well as the balance between the good and the bad. This also applies to eating and fasting. During this fasting, the body utilizes its own fats (the excess fat) to produce energy.

When we eat, our bodies use the energy they require and the excess stored for later use. This is dictated by the presence of the insulin hormone. The increase in the level of insulin during the eating process facilitates the body to store the excess energy by linking it to the long-chain glycogen and then storing them in the liver. Due to the limited space in the liver, some sugar is converted to fat through a process called lipogenesis.

On the other hand, when we are not eating, the insulin within the body decreases and hence signals the body to begin burning the stored energy because the blood glucose level falls during this time.

The easily accessible source of energy during a fast is the glycogen. The compound is broken down into glucose molecules to facilitate the functioning of the body cells. Study indicate that the energy from breaking down glycogen is only capable of driving the body system for about 24-36 hours before the body begins to act on the stored fat as the ultimate source of energy.

It can now be deducted that for healthy living, a state of balance between the fasting and feasting periods is vital. Throughout our lives, it is either we are storing the food or breaking them down. This will mean that there is no weight net gain. Eating from the time we wake up until we go to sleep would lead to the addition of weight since the body acts on the food and further stores the excess. Opting to fast would avert this since more time would be available to burn the stored fat. This should not be an issue since our bodies are designed to work that way.

Factors that hinder one from considering the intermittent fasting.

The evidence-based benefits of intermittent fasting have triggered many to try it for healthy living. However, many factors prevent people from trying this healthy intervention.

A. The fear of being hungry

Regardless of the benefits that come along with intermittent fasting, the body takes much time to adapt and hence the individual. Most people avoid this ancient program because they hate the feeling of being hungry and the discomfort that comes along with the feeling. However, with time your body would have better control over your hunger.

B. Desire for an immediate impact

It is always said that the emotionally strong personalities have patience and optimism in whatever program they engage in. With the belief that this fasting would help you have control over your weight, it is good to remain focused on the diet patterns.

However, the positive effects take much time to manifest (usually three weeks). Most people feel discouraged because of this and end up giving up on it. For example, losing weight with intermittent fasting should not be seen as a race but as the best alternative ever.

C. Fear of losing muscles

Regarding the study by many companies, it is believed that failing to take about 30g of protein after every few hours forces our body to break the muscles as the source of energy.

On the contrary, our bodies are adapted to preserving the muscles even while we are fasting. Again, there is no difference to the body between the proteins taken in a shorter period compared to protein spread throughout the day. This is because protein takes much time before absorption by the body.

In short, it is important to give this program a shot and experience how effectively you would lose weight among other health benefits associated with the program.

Important tricks for effective fasting

- **Never freak out**

It is obvious to be nervous when trying something new. You will ask yourself several rhetorical questions making you eventually change your mind about trying a new idea. This should not be the case when you need to enjoy the health benefits that come with intermittent fasting.

Our body act like a machine and would eventually adapt to the new dieting pattern. Pilon once advised that we should view fasting as a break from eating rather than a period of deficiency.

- **Always stay busy**

It is always said that an idle mind is the devil's workshop. Sitting around thinking about how hungry you are would tempt you into stopping your fast. Engage in activities that would keep you busy to scavenge the thoughts that you are hungry.

Successful applicants of intermittent fasting have their brains always occupied to leave no room for how hungry they are. This would help you overcommit to achieving your desired outcome through fasting.

- **Take zero-calorie drinks**

The main objective of fasting is to allow the body utilize the stored foods for energy. It is, therefore, not advisable to take foods of drinks rich in calories during this period.

Taking beverages like tea and coffee among other drinks that lack calories should be encouraged to avoid dehydration during the fasting process.

- **Never expect miracles**

Intermittent fasting has many roles in our bodies that are not limited to losing extra weight and increasing the insulin sensitivity by our bodies. For the benefits to be experienced, this fasting is just one of the many factors for the desired health benefits. Do not expect to lose about 8% weight simply because you are fasting.

- **Expect discouragements from those around you**

For example, the culture of taking breakfast is so much ingrained to the extent that failing to take it is considered crazy. Most of those around you might try to discourage you against fasting. Having this awareness would be important to help you follow the program to meet your desired health benefits.

- **Regular physical exercise**

Many people see it difficult to go to the gym while fasting not knowing they would be increasing chances for an early achievement of their desired weight. Fasted training can for example result in improved muscle protein synthesis, better metabolic adaptations among other benefits. Have the mentality that fasting would not cause muscle loss during this period.

CHAPTER TWO: History of Intermittent Fasting

Our bodies naturally undergo alternating fasting and feasting. This means that intermittent fasting is part of our livelihood and date back to centuries. I addition to this, even the animals fast as a normal existence course.

For centuries, this fasting has remained effective with the health practitioners, priests, and philosophers using it. For instance, in ancient India and Egypt, voluntary abstaining from food was considered curative, spiritual as well as a preventive intervention against certain conditions.

Since then fasting has remained a religious practice with the Christians, Hindus, Muslims, Taoists, Jainists among other religions.

Christians during the Lent are only allowed to consume the unleavened bread, which was done by Jews long ago during the Pesach or the Passover. During the first two centuries of its existence, fasting was made a voluntary action that entailed receiving the sacraments of the Holy Communion, the ordination of the priests as well as baptism. With time, fasting became an obligation among all Christians. Lenten fast was expanded from its original 40 hours to 4 days with only one meal permitted a day.

Muslims also fast annually during the month of Ramadhan as a form of atonement. They fast from sunrise to sunset during this holy month. Neither food nor fluids are allowed during the fasting period as opposed to many other protocols of fasting. Because of this, they undergo a period of mild dehydration.

The feasting period before sunset and sunrise negates the beneficial effects of this natural therapeutic program because of the increased intake of calories as a result. Considering instructions by the prophet Muhammad, Muslims are also encouraged to fast both on Mondays and on Thursdays of every week.

As a passage of rite, the early man for various important reasons used fasting. Infertility was linked with the anger of the gods and hence fasting was usually done during the autumnal equinoxes to curb the curse. The native Mexicans, as well as the Incas from Peru, also observed fasting to appease their gods.

Historians have come up with publications to illustrate that fasting began a long time ago with our ancestors. Fasting was used to treat the health conditions like the obesity, allergies, high blood pressure and headache among other illnesses.

The ancient Greek historian Herodotus argued that people perceived illness through food. He said that Egyptians were healthy because of their common practice of purification of enemas and vomiting for three days every month.

Plato also realized that fasting was one of the primary treatments. Asclepiad in the 90 BC practiced the use of both the "reorporatsiya" and "metazinkreziya" that entail the use of periodic fasting, bathing, exercising and rubbing.

The ideology of using fasting for health reasons wondered until the middle ages. During this period, people engaged in excessive eating and drinking. This was the reason as to why most of them became severely sick at the age of 40 years. After the miraculous healing of Cornaro, one doctor exclaimed that a strict abstinence from food could help prevent against diseases.

Dr. Chain in the year 1671 to 1743 suggested reforms on the daily diet following recovery from the hell of excessively consuming pork chops and ale.

Today, scientific medicine have become dominant since the drugs were developed. Fasting as a therapeutic intervention fell out of favor in the world. Surprisingly, during this falling out, in Germany, doctors still included the idea of controlled fasting as an integrated medical practice. Dr. Edward Dewey, in the year 1877, was the first person to apply fasting as a mitigation against diseases that involves the loss of appetite and coated tongue. He argued that one should avoid eating once he or she regains his or her appetite and the tongue becomes cleansed for more than 50 days.

However, with the increasing cases of preventable conditions like obesity, several studies have been conducted globally to prove the benefit of fasting in cutting extra weight as well as its psychological effects. Surveillance was done on people with the aim of making a great contribution to the field of science. This led to renewed interest in the reliance in fasting to control the health diseases. Greenfield exclaimed that if people could do a day fast for at least twice a year (one during the spring and one during the autumn), their bodies would mitigate the toxic effects during their daily living.

In support of this natural method, the wide dissemination of therapeutic fasting like the recognized limotherapy further made many health practitioners apply fasting as a medical control practice. Due to this rapid evolution of fasting as a therapeutic intervention in the 21st century, many physicians recommend it for anyone who would wish to have an optimal health regardless of whether he or she is sick or not.

Without forgetting, the hunger strikes experienced among but not limited to the employees against bad leadership.

It is now clear that fasting has remained significant ever since. Fasting has become a means of improving one's health as opposed to the drugs (some with adverse health effects). Most people use fasting as a means of avoiding surgery that might bring complications after that. Let every person develop the belief that fasting among other natural remedies controls the emotions, mental and spiritual aspects of our bodies towards a happy and healthy living.

CHAPTER THREE: Types of Intermittent Fasting

With the research indicating that restricting calories intake is important in increasing the lifespan in humans and other animals, intermittent fasting has been gaining popularity globally for quite some time now. This dieting pattern is not constant in all individual since the health outcomes depend on caloric reduction, hormonal management, decreased hunger as well as the prioritized benefits.

Not taking consideration about how long one stays without eating, intermittent fasting can make one avoid calories intake for between 16 to 36 hours. Further extension of the period over which we fast is what defines this intermittent fasting.

In the mathematical scenario, the vector principle suggests many different routes to the same destination. This is correct when it comes to cutting our bodies off calories for a regulated period. There are different fasting methods that in the end would result in the same health benefits in different people. This is because it is understood that there is no single similarity between two people and that different nutritional approaches would ensure the desired health outcomes are achieved in different individuals.

Each recommended method has its own specific guidelines on what to eat as well as how long our bodies would have to stay without food. It is, therefore, important to choose the best method that you enjoy and believe would work for you.

1. Eat Stop Eat Type of Fasting

This fasting method by Brad Pilon entails avoiding food for up to 24 hours once or twice a week. Just like any other form of fasting, this Eat Stop Eat type of fasting involves eating foods less than what your body is used to. This will, in turn, ensure that the caloric value within the body is cut by a certain percentage.

Most of the fasting techniques require self-discipline in ensuring you achieve the desired outcome. This 24-hour fast, once or twice in every week, however, is flexible since you are the one to decide when to fast as well as when to feast provided it sums to 24 hours of fasting. Opting to fast during your busiest days is the recommended since you do not have time to think about the hunger. The fasting days can as well be adjusted in case of a family event among other planned gatherings to suit your preference.

During this fasting period, only the non-calorific drinks like coffee, tea and water are allowed to protect the body against excessive dehydration. The solid foods are not allowed during this period.

As an important point to note, ensure you normally eat during the feasting time. That is, consume the normal amount of food as if you have not been fasting. Taking more food than normal would render your effort of cutting extra weight useless since you would be experiencing constant undesirable weight gain.

How the 24-hour fasting is done

Just as the name suggests, this type of fasting entails depriving your body of food for a maximum of 24 hours once or twice a week. For example, if you eat today at 8 pm and avoid food until 8 pm the following day, then that is the complete 24-hour fasting technique. Some people might decide to take their meal at 6 am then fast until the following morning. The ultimate outcome would remain the same.

Severe dehydration might occur during this fasting period, and this is the reason why the health practitioners advise us to increase the intake of fluids that are non-calorific to help rehydrate our bodies and as a result avoid the ill effects that might arise from this.

However, just like the other forms of fasting, this 24-hour fasting system remains a challenge to most of the people who would wish to try it for the first time because their bodies are not used to the type of dieting. Some assume that they are entitled to more food during the feasting period because they had fasted. The aforementioned self-control is the virtue that is important in ensuring we all enjoy the benefits of this program.

Research indicate that this is one of the simplest methods we can consider for fasting because once your 24 hours are over, you get back to your normal feeding habit provided you don't overeat.

Advantage of this Eat Stop Eat method of fasting

This type of fasting is one of the most common techniques that people prefer. This is because of some of the advantages that it has recorded over the others.

- **Abstinence from the intake of calories for a longer duration**

Considering most of the fasting forms available, an individual can decide to extend their fasting by just an hour or two. However, this is different with this type of fasting since one has to survive with non-caloric drinks for a longer period of time (24 hours).

This means that with this type of fasting, you lose weight much faster compared to the other forms like the Lean Gain type that requires one only to fast for 14 hours in women and 16 hours in men.

- **This method is easy to adapt**

Fasting is like interfering with the way our bodies operate. It takes our bodies many struggles to work effectively during the fasting period. The 24-hour fasting technique is an easy one since the only rule involved is that one must stay without food for 24 hours.

Unlike most of the fasting types, this method does not limit the amount of food to take during the days you are not fasting. Recent research conducted indicates that this would still ensure a deficit in calories. In addition to this, this Brad's system does not restrict you from taking your favorite foods. This has been a selling factor for this type of fasting.

Compared to some forms that require one to fast for about 36 hours, this Eat Stop Eat strategy is relatively simple, especially for the newbies.

- **This method is flexible**

This point is greatly explained in at the explanatory part of this chapter. This one factor influences how people adopt this fasting technique as a means of losing extra weight among other health benefits.

In this context, flexibility means that you can decide on your favorable time to begin your fast without having to follow the strict orders by the physicians. For example, one decides to begin his or her fasting in the morning or even in the afternoon provided the fasting duration sums to 24 hours.

2. The Alternate-Day Fasting

This type of intermittent fasting requires one to fast on alternating days by either taking fewer calories or none at all to realize its sudden positive effects. This method comes with many versions provided at the end of the day you deny your body food for a specific period. The most common version of this alternate-day fasting involves the 'modified' fasting where one is only allowed to consume only up to about 500 calories counts per fasting day.

Depending on the different people, this form of fasting can involve a person fasting for the whole day or just some hours. Just like illustrated, a full fast is never recommended for those who are trying to fast for the first time.

With this type of fasting, you would be going to be very hungry most of the times a week. This is very unpleasant and might as well have unpleasant effects with time.

This type of intermittent fasting is ideal as a great weight loss instrument and lowering the chances of one getting both the type 2 diabetes and heart conditions.

How to do the alternate-day fasting

Just as the name suggests, you are required to fast for a day then eat whatever you feel like the following day. As a condition in any form of fasting, the only digestible you are required to ingest are the non-caloric beverages like the water and tea among the many others. These are aimed at hydrating our bodies, which constantly dehydrate during the fasting durations.

During the non-fasting periods, you are allowed to eat whatever you desire. This one thing makes this type of fasting a unique and important strategy to ensure your body utilizes the stored energy.

Considering "The Every Other Day," one of the modified ADF strategy, an individual is only required to consume about 25% of his or her general energy requirements. This mostly translates to 500 calories during the fasting days.

Professional nutritionists advise that we include more fruits, vegetables, whole grains, dairy products as well as proteins in our diet during our non-fasting days. This helps our body to be able to have more nutrients to break down during the fasting period the following day.

3. The Warrior Diet as a Fasting Strategy

There are sometimes you feel like eating less during the day and end up eating much at night. This is what The Warrior Diet stands for. Ori Hofmekler was the first to introduce this form of fasting. This form of intermittent fasting was named Warrior diet because of the Warriors' ability to stay up to 20 hours during the day without food and eat a heavy meal during the remaining four hours of the night. With regard to this, the warrior diet entails the undereating during the day that is, fresh juice, raw fruit, few servings of protein as well as vegetable.

This less intake of less food during the day is followed by a heavy meal during the night to help facilitate the body's parasympathetic nervous system in enhancing a calm, relaxed and enhanced digestion.

What you decide to eat and when you are eating it is of great concern when it comes to this type of fasting. It is recommended we begin by consuming vegetables, proteins, and fat in significant quantities. Add carbohydrates in case you still feel hungry. The feasting period must be about four hours.

One unique and important fact about this type of fasting is that it emphasizes on the paleo diet, that is, intake of the unprocessed, whole foods.

According to Hofmekler, the body fats are burnt during the day to produce energy that helps the body produce hormones at night during the heavy feasting.

Benefits of this type of fasting

The fact that this type of fasting allows someone to ingest food in a small amount during the fasting period makes it widely acceptable. This makes it easy to get through unlike the other forms of fasting, which requires one to survive on only the non-caloric drinks or sometimes a dry fast.

During the 20 hours of fasting, the growth hormone is increased and just like any other type of fasting; fewer calories are consumed.

This type of fasting is flexible since, during the four hours of feasting period, the makeup of that food is not important provided adequate protein is consumed. This means that you can as well consume the 'junk' foods and still live a happy and fulfilling life.

In general, having a single meal in a day is economically affordable and hence simple to live by. This, as a result, has led to reduced stress among those who are of less economic status but still desire to drop some weight among the other health benefits of fasting.

Individuals that have tried this type of fasting record increased rates of fat loss as well as the energy levels.

Drawbacks of the warrior diet type of intermittent fasting

Trying to acquire the maximum calories in one meal means that the meal has to be very large that eating would. As a result, lead to discomfort. This fact discourages many people from applying this type of fasting procedure.

Although, it is better since a person is allowed to consume few snacks during the 20 plus fasting hours, following the strict guideline on what needs to be eaten can be hectic to many people.

This fasting form would also cause a headache during planned social gatherings like the family meetings and the wedding ceremonies. It would be tricky for some people to avoid the mouth-watering foods at the expense of just consuming fruits or vegetable.

Other individuals do not have the ability to consume large meals at a time and hence find this type of fasting technique quite discouraging. In addition to this, the following of the strict guideline involved would also not favor their preferences.

4. The 16/8 Method: Fast for 16 hours each day

Martin Berkhan, a fitness expert, popularized this type of fasting.

This type of fasting involves an individual fasting for a maximum of 16 hours with a feasting window of about 8 hours. During the 8 hours, one can have more than one meal depending on their preferences. Women, however, due to their delicate nature, should fast for only a maximum of 14 hours.

Just like any other form of fasting, no consumption of calories is allowed during the fasting period.

Research indicate that most of the users prefer fasting during the night and end up breaking the fast six hours after waking up.

This type of intermittent fasting is ideal and easy for every person provided a specific feeding window is maintained constant. If this is not considered, an undesirable hormone imbalance will result making it difficult to adapt to the new fasting program.

This type of fasting is ideal for the gym-goers. When you work out determines the feeding window. For example, the days you go to the gym requires that you consume more of carbohydrates than fats as compared to increased intake of fats during the resting days. However, the protein intake should remain relatively high every other day depending on gender, body fat, age as well as the desired outcomes of the fast.

Whole, unprocessed foods should consist a larger portion of the meal during the feasting duration. This means that the type of food you eat during the feasting period would determine the general outcome. Eating many junk foods or foods rich in excess calories would not be helpful in achieving your desired weight. Non-caloric drinks like tea and water can be ingested during this fasting window.

Benefits of 16/8 fasting protocol

This type of fasting enhances hormonal management. This is common in all the intermittent fasting programs, but it is far much advanced in this 16/8 fasting procedure. This makes it an ideal program for all.

Within the 8-hour feasting period, you can eat whatever you wish. Taking three meals during the feeding period makes it easy for those who try this type of fasting. For a comfortable and successful fasting, this is one of the best fasting methodologies.

During the fasting periods, the feeling of hunger is a common experience. This is not the case when it comes to this type of intermittent fasting. Recent studies indicate that the 16/8 fasting form has a hunger management advantage. The infrequent meals involved make you feel fuller for a longer period.

Drawbacks of the 16/8 fasting procedure

Unlike the other forms of fasting, this type of fasting is effective when one does workouts in a fasted state. This makes it hectic for those individuals that hate engaging in physical exercises.

The difficulty in following the simple nutrition plans when it comes to this type of fasting forces many people to shift the feasting duration to inconvenient intervals. This also applies to what we eat in relation to the type of activities you engage in during this time.

5. Fat Loss Forever Intermittent Fasting Method

This fasting method is branded a 'hybrid' since it was developed following the combination of all the three most common types of fasting: the Warrior Diet, Eat Stop Eat, and the Lean Gains methods. This was the work of Dan Go and Romaniello to utilize the strengths of every individual fasting methods while ruling out their weaknesses. According to the plan by your professional instructor, a specific intermittent fasting technique is followed on certain days. Until you meet your desired outcomes.

This method is ideal for those who desire to lose more weight within a limited period. This is possible when you engage in this type of fasting for a period of 12 weeks.

It is advisable that you engage in longer fasts on the days that you are very busy since you have no space to think about how hungry you are.

Benefits of Fat Loss Forever IF Method

Since it involves a combination of all the three outstanding fasting methods, this cocktail type of fasting ensures that you achieve your goals within limited time. For the controlled 12-week program, significant outcomes are observed. This is the reason why this type is important for those individuals that are never patient.

Advanced hormonal management. Combining the three types of fasting would increase the concentration of growth hormone within the body and hence the related benefits.

Drawbacks of Fat Loss Forever IF Method

This become a more complicated system to follow for those individuals who are not able to follow the strict guidelines of the individual fasting methods. This is because, during the stipulated duration of the fasting program, each individual fasting method is considered on specific days.

Some people use this type of fasting as an excuse to eat the processed, unwholesome meals. This makes many people not to enjoy the benefits of this Fat Loss Forever IF Method.

In conclusion

With the many types of intermittent fasting, not limited to the once mentioned above, it is important to consult a health professional to help you choose the best strategy that fits you. This would be the first step once you realize that this strategy would simplify your nutrition. This is because people have varying personalities and chemical composition hence different techniques would work for each one of them.

Personal experimentation can also be helpful when it comes to determining the ideal method that fits you. Consider trying each method at different times to ensure you achieve your desired outcome.

It is good to choose the method that makes you comfortable since there is no form of fasting that would produce positive results when you feel miserable and stressed out.

CHAPTER FOUR: Benefits of Intermittent Fasting

This belief that meal skipping leaves our bodies in a starvation mode has proved to be a great challenge in the campaign about fasting as a health remedy for various conditions. This is possible because of the cut calories which allows our body to utilize the stored energy for the normal cell functioning. The benefits of the fasting supplements like the vegetables, nuts, fruits and fish among others make this strategy an important weapon against diseases.

The stigmatization that comes along with this meal skipping tendency has made the health practitioners to avoid as much as possible giving this strategy as an intervention against the health problems. This, however, does not undermine the incredible benefits that come along with this practice. This is because of the mounting evidence that other key aspects of diet (how and when often people eat) play an important role in a healthy lifestyle.

A. Fasting helps in losing extra weight

There are many ways to lose weight. According to different studies, intermittent fasting proves to be one of the ideal ways in losing some extra body mass. This is because the body is allowed to burn the fat cells to produce the energy used within the body. This would not be the case during the normal dieting since the ingested calories would be the ones broken down instead.

To further support the importance of skipped meals on weight loss, this intermittent fasting is known to facilitate the hormone functioning that enhances the loss of weight. That is, reduced calories intake would result in low insulin levels, increased noradrenaline as well as a higher growth hormone levels. This hormone optimization increases the rate at which our bodies act on the body fat to be the ultimate energy source. Fortunately, we end up losing the extra mass thereby achieving our desired weight reading.

Introducing your body to the actual intermittent fasting elevates the body metabolic rate by about 14% to facilitate the fast burning of the body fat. It is clear that this would result in a loss of some pounds of mass.

With the above explanation, it is clear that intermittent fasting is helpful when in need of losing some mass since calories intake is limited. This is also possible due to our boosted metabolic rate.

Research conducted in 2014 indicates that about 8% of weight is lost between 3-24 weeks of intermittent fasting. This important factor has triggered many individuals to try this remedy for a successful venture. This was supported by the loss of about 4-7% loss of the waist circumference indicating that the belly fat responsible for frequent abdominal pain among those with heavy bodies is burnt.

As a caution, this method would not result in loss of weight if you opt to compensate the fasting period by eating much during the non-fasting periods.

B. Intermittent fasting promotes longevity

Though it is difficult to believe, the less you eat, the longer you might live. This is supported by most studies that show a higher life expectancy among those who have the culture of skipping meals than those who enjoy all the meals.

This type of fasting boosts our immunity and the restorative properties of the body. This ensures that we live a longer and enjoyable life with no fear of dying anytime soon.

This was supported by research done on the c. Elegans worm that have some genes that we too have. The research indicated an increased longevity if subjected to similar intermittent fasting conditions.

It is clear that fasting reduces the insulin concentration within the body of an individual. Brain insulin signaling reduction has been seen to further increase the longevity by literally knocking the brain insulin receptor out or by calorie restricting. This is also recognized in rats.

A healthy lifestyle is connected to increased longevity. This means that relying on intermittent fasting has a means of enhancing our health by burning the belly fat, for example, would. As a result, translate to increased longevity.

Aging is associated with a slow rate of metabolism. This means that the younger you look, the higher the metabolism rate. Cutting the introduction of calories within the body would facilitate an increased metabolic process since it takes less time for the little food ingested to be digested. This slows down the aging rate of an individual.

For a long and happy life, it is important to consider this special intervention that has a proven track record from recent studies.

C. Intermittent fasting with heart health

Researchers indicate that heart problem is one of the killer diseases in the world today. In connection to this, the elites argue that the various risk factors are connected to either a decreased or increased chances of heart disease. Such health markers include the blood pressure, the blood triglycerides, the LDL cholesterol and the inflammatory markers among other factors.

However, this intermittent fasting has been proven to harmonize these risk factors for a healthy heart. This is possible because those who fast have control over the amount of calorie they take into their bodies and this then translates to better and healthy heart due to the favorable eating choices.

The rate at which our bodies metabolize the cholesterol within the body determines the heart health. Regular intermittent fasting increases the body metabolic rate. This ensures that the bad cholesterol is broken down as fast as possible to minimize the risks of heart diseases by reducing the risks of gaining extra weight and diabetes.

If you need to begin a fast with the intention of maintaining a healthy heart, consult your personal physician on the types of foods or drinks to use as a supplement during your fasting periods. Maintaining a heart-healthy diet and regular physical exercises further improves the general health.

Lowering the levels of fat within the body because of intermittent fasting lessens the kidney workload hence a lower blood pressure. This lowered blood pressure as well as the increased production of the growth hormone enhances an effective cardiac function.

D. The role of intermittent fasting in the war against cancer

Cancer is a chronic disease that is characterized by the abnormal cell growths. Intermittent fasting, therefore, has been seen as an important arsenal to help in the killing of cancer cells.

During this period, the normal cells 'hibernates' while the cancerous cells continue multiplying trying to find alternative survival means but without any success.

As a common measure against cancer, the normal cells were found to have the ability to withstand the chemotherapy. This therapy is best done when the body is in a starvation mode to easily differentiate the healthy cells from the cancerous ones.

Regardless of its remedy against cancer, intermittent fasting is not a strategy that every cancer patients can rely on. For example, those patients who have lost about 10% of their total body weight or have chronic conditions such as diabetes should not subject themselves to fasting. This can be so disastrous to the health of the individual.

It is, therefore, important to consult your physician to enable you to understand the stage of your condition before turning to fasting as the ultimate intervention against cancer.

E. Fasting improves the immune system

Considering all the health benefits that come along with fasting, it is correct to argue that it boosts our bodies in the fight against diseases. These health effects result when the free radicles are reduced, the cancerous cells starved and the inflammatory condition regulated. These effects only occur when our bodies are in the state of fast.

As an illustration, when an animal is sick it does not feed. This action minimizes the pressure on the internal body system in the war against diseases.

During fasting, a regenerative switch gives an 'OK' for the stem cells to create new white cells. The body, as a result, gets rid of the damaged cells during this period. This entire procedure facilitates the creation of literally a new immune system.

Records indicate that individuals who fast for about four days in every six months experience limited cases of infections.

During this starvation period, the body tries to save energy by recycling the unused or damaged white cells.

F. Health benefits of intermittent fasting for the brain

Since our body organs are interconnected, whatever benefits the body would as well benefit the brain. This, therefore, means that the different types of fasting are beneficial when it comes to brain health.

When subjecting yourself to any form of intermittent fasting, the metabolism rates aimed at reducing the oxidative stress, reducing the blood sugar levels, insulin resistance as well as reduced inflammation. These physiological processes are helpful when it comes to a healthy brain in humans and animals in general.

This fasting increases the levels of the brain-derived neurotrophic factor hormones. The level of this hormone lowers during depression along with other various brain complications. This increase in the level of these hormones indicates that the brain is in its favorable state.

This skipping of meals facilitates the growth of nerve cells within the brain to enhance the brain functioning.

G. Spiritual importance of intermittent fasting

The one thing that most people know is that fasting is a means of losing extra mass to achieve the desired body weight. This is not the case when it comes to religion. Nearly every religion values the role of fasting in bringing them close to their Supreme Being.

In a religious setup, fasting is not necessarily meant for health benefits but as a means of showing faith in your beliefs. Fasting entails saying an 'NO' to the natural appetite to be close to God the Almighty. For example, Muslims fast during the month of Ramadhan as a directive by Prophet Mohamed to enhance their purifications. Christians, Hindus, Puritans among all the other spiritual religions do fast for reasons such as famine or even drought.

The spiritual fasting also helps in discovering the self-awareness of an individual. This is an early and quick track to discover where your addiction and truth lie.

The Side Effects of Intermittent Fasting

Intermittent fasting record both the positive and negative impacts. This depends on the individual hormonal stability as well as the type of fasting method employed.

Any intervention that is introduced comes with its own guiding principles. Acting against these principles would mean you experience the undesirable outcome. This is the same when it comes to all methods of fasting.

I. **Obsession with the feeding and fasting window**

Since intermittent fasting entails alternating periods of fasting and feasting, some individuals tend to get obsessed with when the feasting time would come. They end up thinking about food as a result.

To make this worse, some dieters fail to follow the IF standard guidelines and end up extending their fast period to observe an immediate outcome. In the end, unhealthy weight loss results that is later regained.

The reason why most obsessed dieters regain their weight is that they eventually go back to their old eating habits.

II. **The feeling of starvation**

Food cravings and hunger are some of the usual challenges when someone is trying to cut some mass off for healthy living. Hunger pangs have been observed in some individuals who eat six meals during the non-fasting period.

The feeling of hunger is an early sign when you begin your fasting journey to enjoy the benefits that follow. Your body adapts to the state with a time of regular controlled fasting.

III.   Caffeine addiction

Intermittent fasting allows the consumption of non-caloric beverages to enable the dieters to remain energized and rehydrated. Such drinks include coffee, water, and tea. Both the coffee and tea contain caffeine that is addictive to users. Dieters end up over-relying on the coffee and tea.

Addiction to these drinks is associated with stress, anxiety and poor sleeping habit, which as a result leads to the undesirable regaining of weight.

IV.   Reduces athletic performance

Though it is advisable to engage in lighter exercise during the fasting period to realize faster weight loss, intense workouts have been found to cause injury to the dieter. In addition to this, exercising during the fasting period causes extra fatigue than usual.

V.   Headaches

Due to the stress that we expose our body to during this fasting period, headaches are common experiences. This is the reason why non-caloric drinks are allowed during the fasting region. For example, drinking water was seen to relieve the headaches in some cases.

VI.   Imbalanced hormone in women

Missed periods, early-onset menopause and metabolic disturbances are some of the negative effects that intermittent fasting have on women. This is because women hormones are very sensitive to energy intake. Long fasting hours would, therefore, interfere with the hormones. To curb this, professionals advice that women try the modified form of intermittent fasting (crescendo).

The side effects above are not for a specific type of intermittent fasting. It is, therefore, vital to consult your physicians to help you select the best fasting strategy to lose the extra weight.

CHAPTER FIVE: Women and Intermittent Fasting

With the increased campaign on the role of intermittent fasting as a means of cutting off extra weight among the several other health benefits, it was discovered that women were extremely sensitive to starvation and hence responded differently to this skipping of meals. That is, fasting might result to a hormonal imbalance and hence fertility problems in women if not done correctly. This is the body's way of protecting the fetus (even when we are not expectant). This affects women as young as in their mid-20s.

Scientific studies indicate that prolonged calories deficit, as well as reduced fat mass, might lead to different forms of menstrual dysfunction (amenorrhea) as well as decreased estradiol, insulin and leptin levels among women.

Fasting and the female hormones

In both women and men, hypothalamic-pituitary-gonadal axis acts systematically. The hypothalamus first releases the gonadotropin hormone that in turn triggers the pituitary gland to produce both the follicular stimulating hormone and the luteinizing hormone. Both the LH and the FSH act as gonads (testes in men or ovaries in women). In women, for example, these gonads facilitate the production of both the estrogen and progesterone in women to help in ovulation.

Women, unlike men, experience very specific and regular hormonal cycles. This, therefore, means that the gonadotropin hormones have to be timed to avoid getting the physiological function out of balance. The GnRH are sensitive to environmental determinants including the simple skipping of meals. This, therefore, calls for a gentle and controlled implementation of the intermittent fasting strategy.

The kisspeptin, a protein that is made in the hypothalamus, is responsible for the production of the gonadotropin hormones in both women and men for proper reproductive functions. Because of the more kisspeptin in women than in males, hence a greater sensitivity to insulin, ghrelin and leptin-the hormones that react to satiety and hunger.

The normal signs of a hormonal imbalance when in a starvation mode

1) The feeling of fatigue.

This feeling normally occurs because of respiration in a limited supply of oxygen. Engaging in uncontrolled fasting might affect the normal functioning of the hormones responsible for the breaking down of the accumulated lactic acid within the body tissues.

2) The feeling of depression

This feeling of hopelessness results when you engage in different forms of fasting with no significant outcome. The failure of your body to benefit from fasting is due to the altered normal hormonal balancing.

Among the other signs of an altered hormonal functioning are a headache, irregular periods and bloating.

To curb this, scientists argue that fasting on nonconsecutive days might be useful in maintaining the hormones in check among the women. This is known as the Crescendo type of fasting since you try the different fasting methods until you identify the suitable one that matches your body system.

The crescendo intermittent fasting for women

Jumping into intermittent fasting for the women can be very hard due to their characteristic hormone fluctuating levels. It is, therefore, important for the newbies to consider a modified intermittent type of fasting (crescendo).

This type of fasting requires that a woman fasts on nonconsecutive days. The hormones do not go frenzy when one applies this type of meal skipping.

The modified fasting technique is a more gentle approach in ensuring the women adapt to fasting. Done right, this can be a great remedy in ensuring you lose some extra mass without altering the hormonal balance as a result.

Though Crescendo type of fasting is not necessary for all women, it can be successful when some of the following rules are taken into consideration.

 ➢ **Skip meals for about 2-3 nonconsecutive days.**

Professionals advise that during the fasting days, the woman engages herself for about sixteen hours. It is also important to engage in physical exercise during the fasting period. The exercise should be less intense.

> ### Drink non-caloric beverages during the fasting period

During this fasting period, the amount of calories taken is cut to allow the body utilize the stored fats for energy. Non-caloric drinks such as water, tea, and coffee among others should be consumed to rehydrate the body after dehydration during this fasting period.

> ### Eat normally when under a high-cardio day

When engaging in heavy training, one can be tempted to compensate the lost energy by eating more food than he or she eats on the normal days. This helps the body adapt to the starvation state with time.

> ### Add an additional fasting day

After about two weeks of fasting, when you feel comfortable, it is good to extend your weekly fasting by a day to help the body get used to the starvation mode as quick as possible. This is optional depending on the desires of the woman who needs to experiment this special fasting strategy.

> ### Taking about 8 grams of BCAAs during your fasting period

The BCAAs amino acid supplement contains fewer calories that remain vital in providing the energy for the muscle development. This is also helpful in edging off the feeling of hunger or fatigue during this period. Though it is also optional, supplementing your body with these amino acids protects the muscles from being burnt down during this fasting period.

➢ **When to stop fasting**

In case you notice any sign of hormonal imbalance, for example, irregular menstrual cycles or sometimes the eating disorders, stop the fasting immediately. This could mean that the common intermittent fasting is not recommended for you. This is, however, never the case if the procedure is done gently and professionally.

This Crescendo style of fasting is recommended for the women who react adversely to the other forms of fasting. For our women to remain healthy during their fasting periods, it is important to engage in this modified intermittent fasting technique.

CHAPTER SIX: Intermittent Fasting and Caloric Restriction

With the desire to live a longer and happy life, many individuals have turned to reducing the amount of food let into their bodies. This is done professionally to avoid malnutrition. This is what is termed as the caloric restriction. In detail, this caloric restriction entails reducing the total calories count by about 30% to 40% the standard daily requirement. This calories restriction is not fun for either humans or other animals.

Intermittent fasting, on the other hand, involves staying for extra durations without having any food. This can be considered the latest form of caloric restriction strategies since an individual willingly decides to avoid eating for some specific period to experience some of its health benefits. This means that one who subjects himself or herself to intermittent fasting would ultimately lengthen his or her life. There are many different forms of intermittent fasting to choose from.

Similarities between Intermittent Fasting and Calories Restrictions

Just like mentioned above, Intermittent fasting is one of the most recent forms of calories restrictions, if not the most recent. This means that both the CR and IF have some similar principles that define them.

a) Both of them undergo the fasting and feasting periods

Just like the intermittent fasting, caloric restriction involves feeding at the specific period as well as starving for some period. For example, after long hours of hunger, those under caloric restriction tend to eat much food. Feeding once in a day when under the CR, is equivalent to having fasted for about 24 hours each day.

b) They are both aimed at enhancing a longer life

Studies indicate that the fat tissues have an indirect connection with a longer life. The CR's principle desire to increase longevity forces it to, therefore, act on the adipose tissues in order to reduce the fat content.

This is similar to intermittent fasting, which allows the body to burn the stored fats as the alternative source of energy. This reduced fat mass would result in a life-extending effect among those under the program.

c) The importance of physical exercise

The common mouse, the most preferred specimen for scientific studies, does not die of similar diseases as humans. This brings a lot of concern on further studies to exhaust all the factors linked with mortality.

Physicians, as a result, observed that engaging in regular exercises when under restricted calories intake has a synergistic effect on both the inflammation and insulin. Physical exercise, however, would be important in ensuring a longer and healthy life.

d) Both of them involve the feeling of hunger

Caloric restriction just like intermittent fasting alternates the feasting and fasting periods. During the period when you are not eating, the feeling of hunger dominates your body system. What is entailed during this starving period is now what differentiate between the CR from the IF. For instance, in intermittent fasting, drinking of non-caloric beverages is allowed during the fasting period whereas, in other caloric restriction strategies, one is expected to avoid any meal or drinks until the feasting time comes.

e) Both the IF and the CR protect the body against diseases

Increased accumulation of fat within the body tissues is linked to lifestyle conditions such as obesity. These diseases lower the quality of life. This might also lead to mortality, which is against the main principles of both the intermittent type of fasting and calories restrictions. The aim of the two programs is to reduce the amount of fat within the body, therefore, protecting the body against ailments.

Reasons Why Intermittent Fasting Is More Important Than the Calories Restriction Program

Despite the fact that both the strategies are aimed at ensuring life-extension, there must be some specific components that make the two strategies different. The two strategies work differently to ensure they achieve their individual goals of a long and healthy life. For example, caloric reduction entails both the decreased metabolism and the increased appetite while the intermittent fasting, however, involves both the increased metabolism and decreased appetite.

Comparing the two programs, researchers indicate that intermittent fasting is more reliable, in your quest to lengthen life, than the caloric restriction due to several factors.

✓ Intermittent fasting lacks many side effects

Although caloric restriction has the benefit of lengthening the life, it depletes the growth, thyroid and insulin hormones. This CR also manifests as poor cardiac health as well as reducing fertility and libido.

However, intermittent fasting when controlled results in achievement of your desired weight among other health benefits. Your safety is only guaranteed when you choose the best intermittent fasting methods available. It is, therefore, important to visit your physician to guide you through the whole program successfully.

✓ Provides similar metabolic benefits to caloric restriction

Like explained earlier, both the intermittent fasting and caloric restriction programs aim at lengthening life. In geography, the vector principle states that different routes might lead to the same destination. The counselors, however, advise that you choose the best between the two strategies: CR and IF in your quest to achieve a life-extension.

Intermittent fasting, which lacks many negative effects is the best of the two to achieve your desire. Do not end up solving a problem while causing a new one. Consider the IF over the CR for healthy living.

✓ **Intermittent fasting provides an additional metabolic boosting**

Intermittent fasting, in addition to losing weight, protects the body against metabolic damages. This will ensure that all the nutrients are utilized to produce energy for the basic metabolism.

✓ **Intermittent fasting is easily manageable than caloric restriction**

The ultimate goals of both the IF and CR are to lengthen life. Intermittent fasting, however, has easy-to-follow guidelines in ensuring you meet your set target. For example, it is advisable to take non-caloric drinks such as water and tea to rehydrate your body during the fasting period.

In general

Intermittent fasting is a form of caloric restriction that is aimed at ensuring life-extension. The two programs use different principles to attain the same results. This, therefore, means that there is no difference between the two programs.

CHAPTER SEVEN: FAQS about Intermittent Fasting

Intermittent fasting has gained popularity globally due to the evidence-based health benefits that come along with it. To understand better what it entails, many questions have been asked by the lovers of this fasting program. This chapter tries to identify some of the frequently asked questions and provide the relevant responses.

1. What does this intermittent fasting entail?

This program gives the body time to utilize the extra energy it stored. The main principle behind this eating pattern is to allow the body to undergo through alternating fasting and feasting cycles to cut the intake of calories as a result.

2. What is the difference between intermittent fasting and caloric restriction?

The CR and the IF tend to share some principles making it difficult for people to distinguish them. Both focuses on the need to lower the intake of calories to enhance a longer and healthy life.

Intermittent fasting is a form of caloric restriction that is controlled.

3. How do I get started?

Several methods of intermittent fasting have been proven to work effectively as weight-loss tools. Some of the fasting methods include but not limited to the following:

- ❖ The Warrior Diet - involving taking a single meal daily
- ❖ Lean Gains - this involves fasting for about 16 hours then break your meals between the feasting duration of 8 hours.
- ❖ Eat Stop Eat - this is a 24-hour fasting either once or twice in every week.
- ❖ An alternate-day fasting – this involves engaging in fasting on alternating days.
- ❖ The Fast-5 Method – this type entails an individual taking 5 hours between their meals.

To get started. Therefore, it is important to consult professionals and choose the best method that benefits you since each method works well in different people.

4. Who can benefit from intermittent fasting?

With the associated benefits that come along with this program, different types of individuals can adapt to the intermittent program. You should be able to enjoy the outcome provided your professional dietician makes you choose the method that fits you.

5. Am I allowed to eat what I want during the feasting period?

After a long duration of fasting, it is good to eat normal as if you were not fasting. Avoid trying to compensate the fast by eating more than you are used to. This normally depends on an individual's lifestyle regarding your daily energy expenditure and food preference and quality. Many individuals need a larger amount of calories to sustain them during the 16-hour fast than for example if you are fasting less than 16 hours. That also depends on your purpose of intermittent fasting such as rapid body weight loss or if you are practicing fasting for spiritually reasons.

6. Can I drink water during my fasting period?

The main aim of this type of fasting is to reduce or cut down the intake of calories to force the body to break down its energy reservoir preferably excess body fat to be the ultimate energy source. During this time, the body can become extremely dehydrated.

Therefore, drinking water among other non-caloric beverages such as tea and coffee are allowed to help in the body's rehydration. However, you need to be careful with coffee and other drinks that contain caffeine since they are diuretics meaning they make you urinate more frequently causing more loss of body fluid thus making you thirsty.

7. Is intermittent fasting advisable for the weightlifters?

Having in mind that fasting breaks down the excess fat within the body to achieve a leaner body and healthier lifestyle, engaging in regular physical exercises such as strength training would further facilitate the burning of fat stored within the body system and maintain or even possible gain muscle tissue.

8. Is it good to have a cheat day?

Some fasting methods such as the 8-hour Diet for seven days is difficult to follow hence up to four cheats in a week is acceptable. These cheat days can work for you, but you should be careful to avoid these cheats since they can lessen the effect of intermittent fast benefits.

9. Can fasting lead to muscle loss?

This should not worry you much since the different methods of intermittent facilitate the breaking down of fats and not the muscles. This would only work when you fully have control of the fasting program. To prevent or minimize muscle loss you should be eating high-quality foods (fats, protein, and carbohydrates) preferably animal based food if you are not a vegan. That way when you start your fasting cycle your body and in particular your muscles are nourished with a complete profile of amino acids from animal based protein. The other components are adding strength workout during the intermittent fasting and doing the strength workout at the end of the IF, so when you break up the fast, you can replenish your muscle tissues with glycogen, protein, and fats.

10. What happens when you fast for 3 days in a raw?

Alternate-day fasting discourages against fasting for consecutive days. However, depending on your lifestyle and preference, there are no ill effects on skipping meals for three or more successive days.

11. Can I take snacks during my fasting period?

The feelings of thirst and hunger develop in the hypothalamus. Either of the feelings can be so tempting during the fasting period. In the case of this, just like mentioned earlier, consider filling your belly with non-caloric beverages such as limewater, hot tea or even coffee.

12. Is intermittent fasting a form of starvation?

Starvation means an extreme malnutrition due to a deficiency in caloric intake within the body. This can be so disastrous to the general health of an individual. In intermittent fasting, however, calories are stored within the body in the form of fat to produce sufficient energy to the body when broken down.

13. Who is not advisable to practice intermittent fasting?

Although IF has been practiced by humans for millennia and very possible, it is part of our human evolution since our ancestor's hunters, and gatherers did not have a stable and guaranteed amount of foods during the different seasons. However, it is advisable not to practice fasting if you are:

-Pregnant since you need to nourish yourself and the baby thus it is not a good time to do that.

-Breastfeeding is very taxing on the mom's body beside the baby needs all the possible nourishment that comes from mom.

-Individuals who have a high amount of stress due to many reasons such as work project completion and other unfortunate situations that are causing a high amount of stress. Your body most likely needs as much help from nutrition at this time. Therefore, it is not advisable to fast.

-Individuals with certain health disorders such as diabetes and other health concerns should consult with their qualified health practitioners and see if intermittent fasting be practiced or not.

CHAPTER EIGHT: Conclusion

Because of the health effects that come along with the stored fat within the body tissue, researchers worked hard to come up with strategies to burn them as the source of fuel within the body. Limiting the calories intake into the body meant that the body had to work on the stored fats to facilitate the basic metabolism. This is a caloric restriction. As a form of caloric restriction, intermittent fasting (an eating pattern that alternated the fasting period and the feasting period) has recently become common in the fight against lifestyle conditions like obesity.

Fasting is a historic process since our ancestors fasted because they either lacked food or for religious reasons. Without knowing, our bodies undergo fasting when we are asleep. In addition to this, the moment we are not eating, we are fasting. This, therefore, means that fasting is a natural process vital for our daily survival.

There are many forms of intermittent fasting that work well with different people: Eat Stop Eat, Alternate-Day Fasting, The Warrior Diet, The 16/8 Methods and Fat Loss Forever. Each intermittent fasting technique works well with different individuals and hence the need to consult professionals before selecting the fasting methodology that would be of help to your health.

Women, for example, experiences frequent hormonal imbalance and hence a modified type of intermittent fasting (crescendo fasting) is the most preferred.

Supplementation like the taking of non-caloric beverages during the fasting period is necessary to rehydrate the body.

A number of benefits come with the correct identification of the most favorable form of fasting. Such include both the spiritual and health benefits. The main aim of fasting is to lose the extra weight hence ensuring a long and healthy living. In addition to this, strong immunity is connected to a successful fasting program.

If not done correctly, fasting can have many adverse effects such as heartburns, headaches, frequent diarrhea and infertility among the many others. Engaging in any fasting program, therefore, requires knowledge of the best method of meal skipping as well as how to do it right for the realization of positive outcomes.

With the global spreading of intermittent fasting as a tool of losing some extra weight, there are many concerns that have arisen from the lovers. This book provides responses to some of the most common questions that are asked for a better understanding of this form of caloric restriction.

Therefore, to record positive results out of the fasting program, consult professionals and choose the best strategy that ensures maximum output. Stay healthy by cutting down the intake of calories.

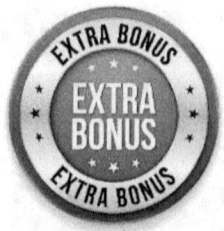 # Chapter

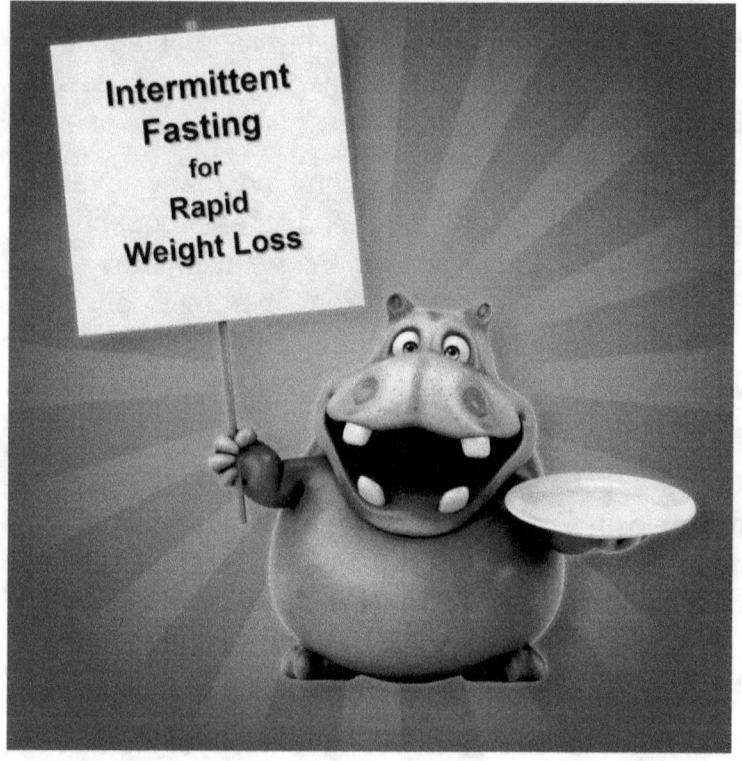

Specific Weight Loss Program Utilizing Intermittent Fasting

As I shared with you in this book, there are different benefits from practicing intermittent fasting however in this chapter I am going to share with you how to optimize your chance to lose weight and specifically body fat while you are practicing IF.

Losing weight can happen almost effortlessly during intermittent fasting practice nevertheless that does not happen with everyone who practices IF unfortunately for various reasons. Although I can't guarantee a hundred percent that you will lose weight and have the same results that I had. But I will share with you effective strategies that you can follow and hopefully you will see noticeable results in few weeks and convert you to an IF believer sooner than later.

Strategy One: Intermittent Fasting with Ketogenic or Low carb/high-fat meals

Some individuals eat meals that are high in carbohydrates and low in fat and possibly low in protein as well. Switching to Keto diet or even low-carb meals might be more effective in making your body to use body fat (ketones) as energy, and gradually but surely you will start to shed off the excess body fat and maintain your muscle tissue.

If you are interested in learning more about ketogenic or low-carb diets you can get my book, All About Ketogenic Diet and will teach you about this topic and how to go about it.

Following Ketogenic diet is stricter than a low-carb diet since you want to force your body to use ketones. When you consume keto diet, your liver will convert fat into ketone bodies and fatty acids.

And likely you will improve the body cells to become less insulin resistance. One possible reason is that you are not bombarding your body with so many carbohydrates (particularly the highly processed ones), leading to, too much insulin secretion, and eventually your cells become resistant to insulin except fat cells.

Another reason for the Ketogenic diet is that can be more satiating due to the high content of fat and moderate amount of proteins which can lead to being satisfied and eating less amount of food and calories. Combine that with intermittent fasting, and you will have a very effective strategy for rapid weight loss.

Examples of Ketogenic and low-carb foods with Pictures

The below images will give you an idea what types of foods to eat and to integrate with your intermittent fasting in order to achieve rapid weight loss outcome.

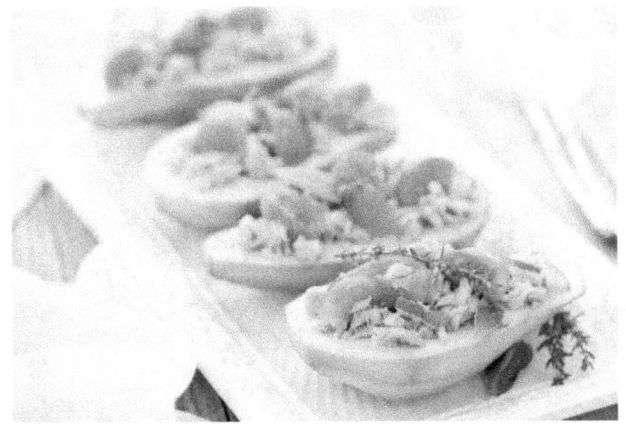

Figure 1 Avocado tuna and tomato salad

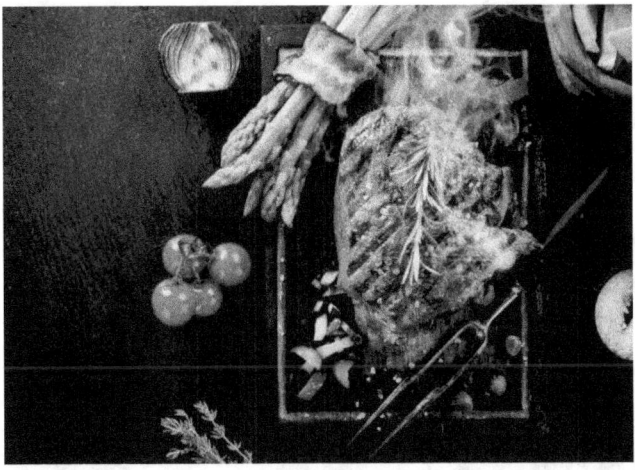

Figure 2 Beef steak with low Starchy Vegetables

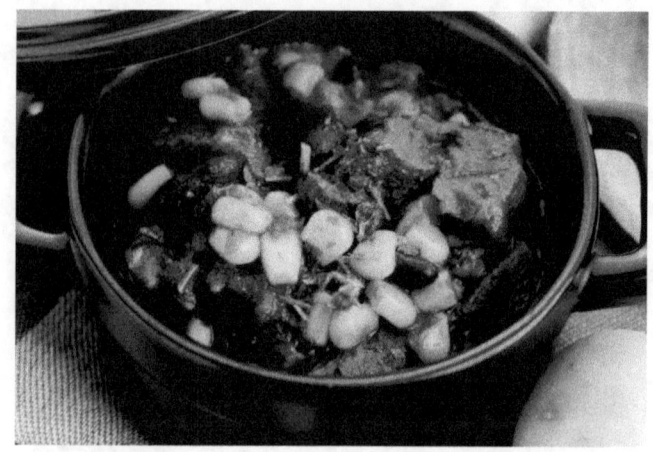

Figure 3 Beef Stew with Vegetables or Beans

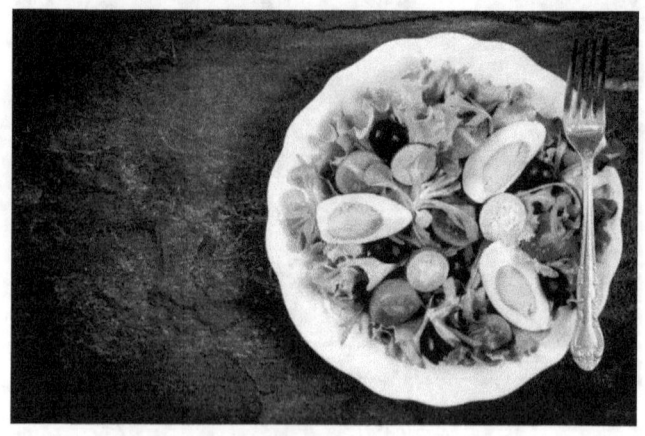

Figure 4 Boiled eggs salad

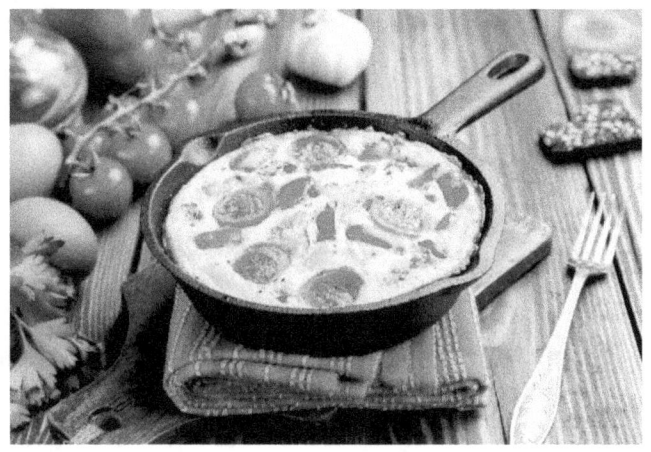

Figure 5 Cheese Bacon Tomato Frittata Keto diet

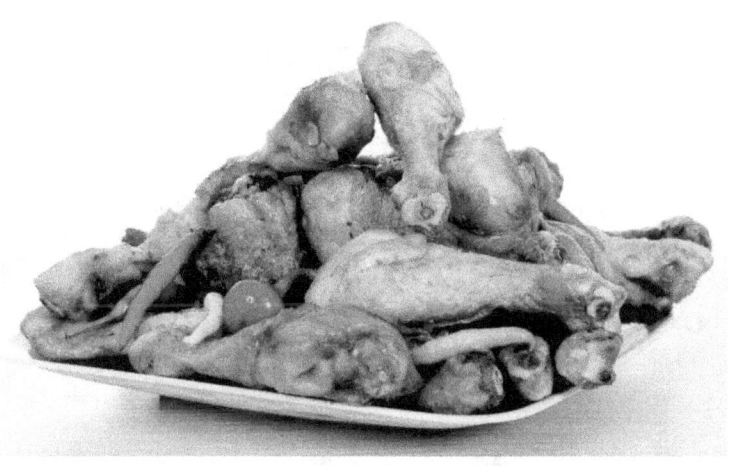

Figure 6 Chicken Drumsticks with sour cream dip

Strategy Two: Resistance Training with Intermittent Fasting

For this strategy, you include a type of resistance training to see rapid weight loss results during intermittent fasting. However, timing is critical here where you want to perform your resistance training at the end of your fasting period.

So if you are fasting for 16 hours, then I would recommend you exercise the last hour or two-hour period.

Fasting = 16 hours	Exercising During the 15th or 16th hour

I performed my resistance training like that for few reasons:

1-I am more likely to use ketones (body fat) since I have been fasting for many hours and I am almost at the end of my fasting cycle.

2-Once I am done with my resistance training, I am soon going to feast or break my fast and replenish my muscles with desperately needed nutrients. Therefore, I am preserving my muscle tissue or even gaining some more, and I have used body fat as energy to workout.

3-It is no fun to perform resistance training, and after you have completed your workout, you still have many hours to wait before completing your intermittent fasting, trust me on that.

Aerobics vs. Resistance Training vs. HIIT During IF

As you have noticed, I mentioned performing resistance training and not aerobics or cardio since it did not yield good results for my clients and me and in particular the female clients. Your resistance workout can be performed at the gym if you like but it can also be done at home with no issues what so ever,

You can also perform High-Intensity Interval Training which is known as HIIT (pronounced as "hit.") and possibly can see even better results than resistance training, but in my experience, that was not necessary, and for many individuals, the HIIT type of training can be very challenging during intermittent fasting.

The idea of including resistance training is to stimulate muscle growth and burn fat using ketone bodies during the fasting period. And the sweet thing here is you will replenish your muscles with some glycogen, fatty acids, and amino acids soon enough since your about a few minutes away from breaking your intermittent fasting.

How to Effectively Perform Resistance Training from Home

Many people think that they have to get a gym membership and use the gym exercise machines to have an effective workout, that's not true for the average person and even beyond the average person. However, this book and this bonus are focused on IF and how to lose bodyweight fast so I will provide you with some exercise names and you can search for them on youtube or the internet. But trust me, these bodyweight exercises can be very demanding, and at the same time, you can adjust them to suit your fitness level.

- All types of pushups (There are at least five varieties I can think of)
- Bodyweight squats
- Lunges
- Pullups
- The good old jumping jack exercise
- The Bear crawl
- Climbing or hiking an uphill for outdoors
- Climbing the stairs in your house
- Step-up exercise
- The walkout exercise
- Sprinting for outdoors training
- Using Resistance bands or tubes at home for pull-down or pull-in
- Resistance tubes for Core exercises

Here you go, try one of the strategies and see which one will work more effectively for you regarding rapid body weight loss during your intermittent fasting and stay with it for as long as you wish. I do however advise that you take a break from doing both at the same time, the IF and Resistance Training or HIIT to give yourself a mental and physical break.

Finally, if you enjoyed this book, please take the time to share your thoughts and post a review on Amazon. It would be greatly appreciated! Thank you and good luck!

www.ingramcontent.com/pod-product-compliance
Lightning Source LLC
Chambersburg PA
CBHW060220290526
45789CB00003B/1347